MUMMIES

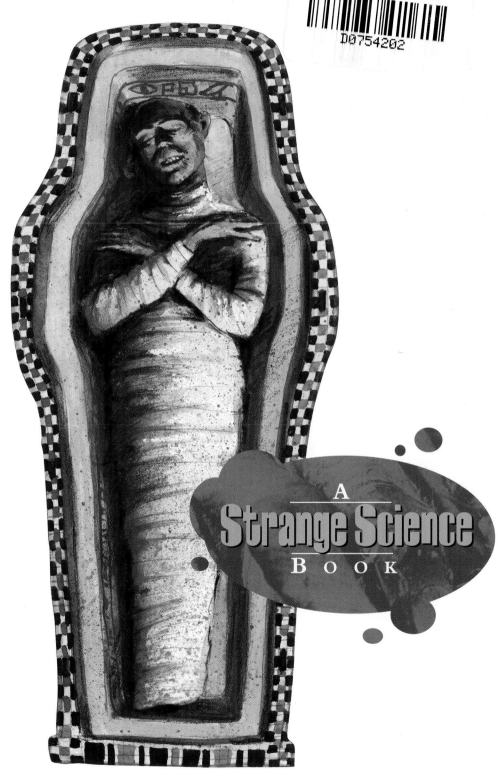

Sylvia Funston

Illustrations by Joe Weissmann

Owl Books are published by Greey de Pencier Books Inc.
70 The Esplanade, Suite 400, Toronto, Ontario M5E 1R2

The Owl colophon is a trademark of Owl Children's Trust Inc.
Greey de Pencier Books Inc. is a licensed user of trademarks of Owl Children's Trust Inc.

Distributed in the United States by Firefly Books (U.S.) Inc.
230 Fifth Avenue, Suite 1607, New York, NY 10001

We acknowledge the financial support of the Canada Council for the Arts, the Ontario Arts Council, and the Government of Canada through the Book Publishing Industry Development Program (BPIDP) for our publishing activities.

Dedication
To Sara from her favorite Mummy.

Cataloguing in Publication Data

Funston, Sylvia
      Mummies

"A strange science book"
Includes index.
ISBN 1-894379-03-9 (bound)
ISBN 1-894379-04-7 (pbk.)

1. Mummies — Juvenile literature.   I. Weissmann, Joe, 1947– .   II. Title.

GT3340.F86   2000   j393'.3   C00-930699-4

Design & art direction: Word & Image Design Studio Inc.
Illustrations: Joe Weissmann

Photo credits
Photos on pages 4, 24, ©1998 David Liittschwager & Susan Middleton; 5, 10, 12, J. Newbury/Sygma; 7, 16, ©Johan Reinhard; 8, Corbis Sygma; 14, ©Silkeborg Museum, Denmark; 20, ©Eric Simonson/Liaison Agency; 21, Dr. Owen Beattie, University of Alberta; 26, 36, 36 inset, courtesy of Royal Ontario Museum, ©ROM; 30, Griffith Institute Ashmolean Museum, Oxford; 32–33, ©Marc Deville/Liaison Agency; 34–35, A.D.P.F./Sygma ©Musée de l'Homme, CL. J. Oster.

Printed in Hong Kong

A   B   C   D   E   F

Contents

DEAD Serious

Imagine you are striding along a mountain pass on a summer day. All of a sudden, you see something sticking out of the melting snow—the head and shoulder of a dead man! Was he a climber who fell and was buried in the snow? Or is an even older mystery being revealed? And what does it have to do with mummies?

Believe it or not, many mummies have been discovered accidentally like this—some in the Alps and Andes mountains; some in deserts in China and Chile; some in bogs in Europe. When you think of mummies, you probably picture cloth-wrapped bodies preserved in Egypt. But not all mummies were created by people. Nature has been preserving bodies much longer—and often more successfully—than we have.

This book is about dead serious stuff, so it includes some things you might not want to raise at the dinner table. It covers 7000 years, or seven millennia, of mummy making. The charts on the opposite page tell you whether nature or people made the mummies in the book. Check the timeline on page 38 to see what was happening around the world while all this mummifying was going on.

Don't forget that mummies were once people with families and lives. Some died naturally, others were sacrificed to gods. Some became mummies by accident; many were mummified deliberately. No wonder mummies are amazing—and a little scary, too.

Cherchen Man (opposite page, left) was mummified by the natural conditions where he was buried. The Chinchorro people preserved the bodies of their dead, including babies (opposite page, right) and children (above).

4

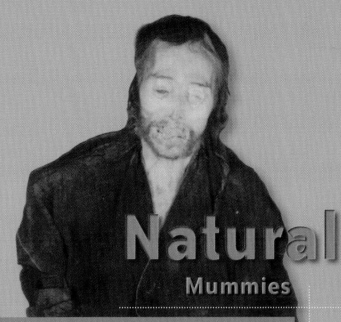

Natural
Mummies

THE ICEMAN
3300 BC (The Alps)

TARIM BASIN MUMMIES
between 2000 BC and 300 BC (China)

BOG BODIES
between 400 BC and AD 400 (Northern Europe)

INCA MUMMIES
between AD 1000 and AD 1500 (The Andes)

MALLORY/IRVINE EXPEDITION
1924 (Mount Everest)

Mummies Made by
People

CHINCHORRO MUMMIES
between 5050 BC and 1500 BC (Chile)

EGYPTIAN MUMMIES
between 3100 BC and AD 400 (Egypt)

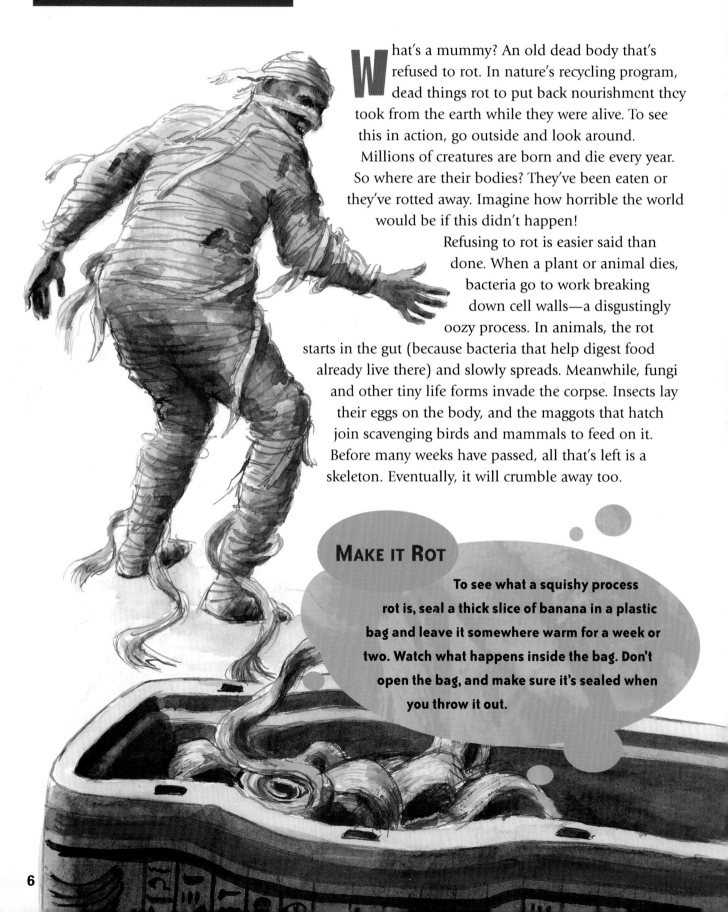

Stop the ROT!

What's a mummy? An old dead body that's refused to rot. In nature's recycling program, dead things rot to put back nourishment they took from the earth while they were alive. To see this in action, go outside and look around. Millions of creatures are born and die every year. So where are their bodies? They've been eaten or they've rotted away. Imagine how horrible the world would be if this didn't happen!

Refusing to rot is easier said than done. When a plant or animal dies, bacteria go to work breaking down cell walls—a disgustingly oozy process. In animals, the rot starts in the gut (because bacteria that help digest food already live there) and slowly spreads. Meanwhile, fungi and other tiny life forms invade the corpse. Insects lay their eggs on the body, and the maggots that hatch join scavenging birds and mammals to feed on it. Before many weeks have passed, all that's left is a skeleton. Eventually, it will crumble away too.

MAKE IT ROT

To see what a squishy process rot is, seal a thick slice of banana in a plastic bag and leave it somewhere warm for a week or two. Watch what happens inside the bag. Don't open the bag, and make sure it's sealed when you throw it out.

The Deadest City on Earth

If you lived in an Italian city called Palermo about 100 years ago, you would visit your dead relatives in its underground cemetery, or catacombs. You'd find their dried-out bodies stretched out in their burial clothes on shelves in the wall, or in coffins with hinged lids. About 6000 bodies lie preserved in the dry, cool air of the catacombs. The city of the dead is still there today, deep below the city of the living.

What's a Mummy and What's Not?

To qualify as a mummy, a dead body must at least have its bones, skin and hair, and it has to look like a human being. Some mummies still have muscles and internal organs, others are padded to look as if they do. A skeleton isn't a mummy, and neither is a fossil whose cells have all changed into stone.

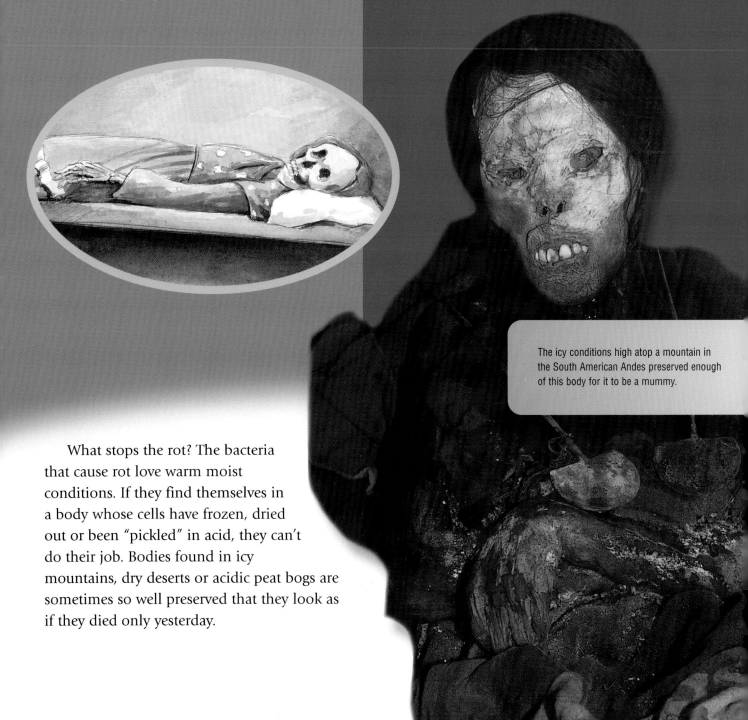

The icy conditions high atop a mountain in the South American Andes preserved enough of this body for it to be a mummy.

What stops the rot? The bacteria that cause rot love warm moist conditions. If they find themselves in a body whose cells have frozen, dried out or been "pickled" in acid, they can't do their job. Bodies found in icy mountains, dry deserts or acidic peat bogs are sometimes so well preserved that they look as if they died only yesterday.

The ICEMAN

The Iceman died 5300 years ago in the Alps, making him the oldest naturally preserved human body found so far.

A Mossy Mystery

Scientists found more than 30 types of mosses clinging to the Iceman's clothes. Nine of them grow in the Italian lowlands south of the mountain pass where he was found, so maybe he came from there. Why so many mosses? Maybe they were used for packing, or for extra insulation. But most likely, like the Romans 3000 years later, the Iceman used the mosses as toilet paper.

One September day in 1991, a group of hikers discovered the body of a man high in the Alps where Austria meets Italy. At first they thought it was the body of a missing climber. When the body was examined carefully, however, the world discovered the extraordinary truth about this mountain climber. He died 5300 years ago. That qualifies him as the world's oldest fully preserved human ever found.

The Iceman died carrying the things he needed for a journey through the mountains. He gives us a rare glimpse into everyday life in Europe at a time when Egyptian mummy-makers were just beginning to practice their bandaging skills. But it was nature that preserved the Iceman's body—the icy conditions high in the mountains froze even the moist inside bits of the body, which usually rot first.

Trekking Checklist

The Iceman was well-equipped for outdoor life. See the list of the gear found with him, below. He knew about wind chill, preventing heat loss from his head and how to protect his toes from frostbite. But some of his things are not so easily explained—the unfinished bow and broken arrows remain a 5000-year-old mystery.

- Fur hat worn fur-side in
- Strap fastener under the chin
- Windproof cape of woven grass
- Deerskin coat
- Leather belt
- Leather pouch containing flint tools and kindling
- Leather loincloth
- Garters to hold up animal-skin leggings
- Calfskin shoes filled with grass
- Yew bow 2 m (6 feet) long, unfinished
- Flint knife in string sheath
- Copper axe with leather-bound yew handle
- Birchbark container for embers to start fire
- Leather and hazelwood rucksack
- Leather and hazelwood quiver containing two bowstrings and 14 broken arrows

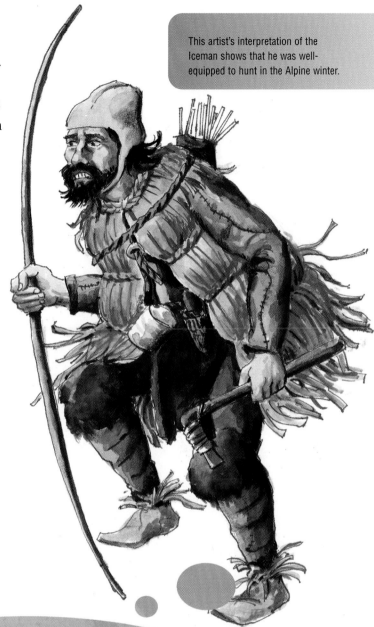

This artist's interpretation of the Iceman shows that he was well-equipped to hunt in the Alpine winter.

MUMMY IN THE FREEZER

To see what icy mountain conditions did to the Iceman's body, you'll need some leftover meat stew (or pet food), a small plastic container with an airtight lid—and patience. Half fill the container with stew; weigh it and write the weight on the container. Seal it and pop it in the freezer. Check it once a week. The moisture will come out of the meat and form ice crystals on top. When there's a thick layer of ice crystals, scrape it off and reweigh the shrivelled meat in the container. Was enough moisture sucked out to make a difference to the weight?

A Chinese RIDDLE

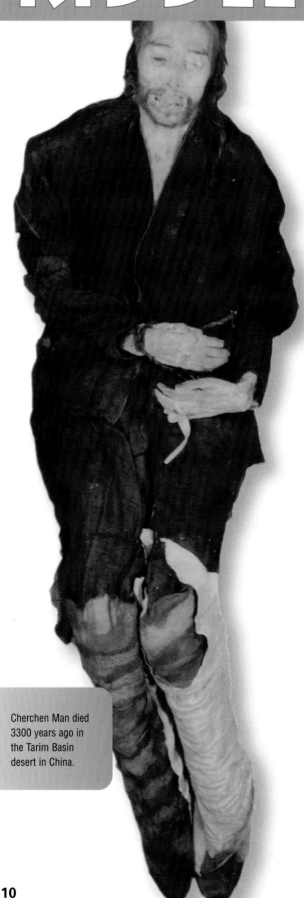

Cherchen Man died 3300 years ago in the Tarim Basin desert in China.

I n a museum, men heave a thick Plexiglass cover off a dead body. As a sickly sweet smell fills the air, a technician pulls up her face mask and looks for signs of decay. When she nods to a group of foreign photographers, they have only a few minutes to snap pictures before the airtight cover is lowered into position again.

Why journey to the treacherous Taklamakan Desert in China's Tarim Basin to take pictures of a dead man? Well . . . the body is 3300 years old, perfectly preserved and alien to this part of the world. Cherchen Man, as the mummy is known, is taller than most Asians, has light brown hair, a bushy beard, deep-set round eyes and a big nose. So what was this European-looking person doing in a remote region of Asia, long before trade caravans travelled the Silk Road between China and Europe? Whatever it was, he wasn't doing it alone.

More than 100 mummies just like Cherchen Man have been discovered in the Tarim Basin. Buried over a span of 1700 years, they're all better preserved than any Egyptian mummy from then. Why? They were buried in bottomless coffins placed in desert salt beds. The best preserved bodies were probably buried in winter, so they would have chilled rapidly. The salty sand then sucked moisture out of the bodies so fast, they dried out before they could begin to rot.

It's thought that ancient Chinese civilization developed for thousands of years without being influenced by other nations. Yet the Tarim mummies prove that outsiders were living in China 4000 years ago. Where did these travellers come from, and did they introduce new ideas into China?

• DNA tests of your cells can tell who you're related to. Early results from DNA tests on some Tarim Basin mummies indicate that they were related to people from central Europe. But it's possible that others might have links with Persia (now Iran). One male mummy had a tattoo on his face that looks like the symbol of Mithras, the Persian sun god.

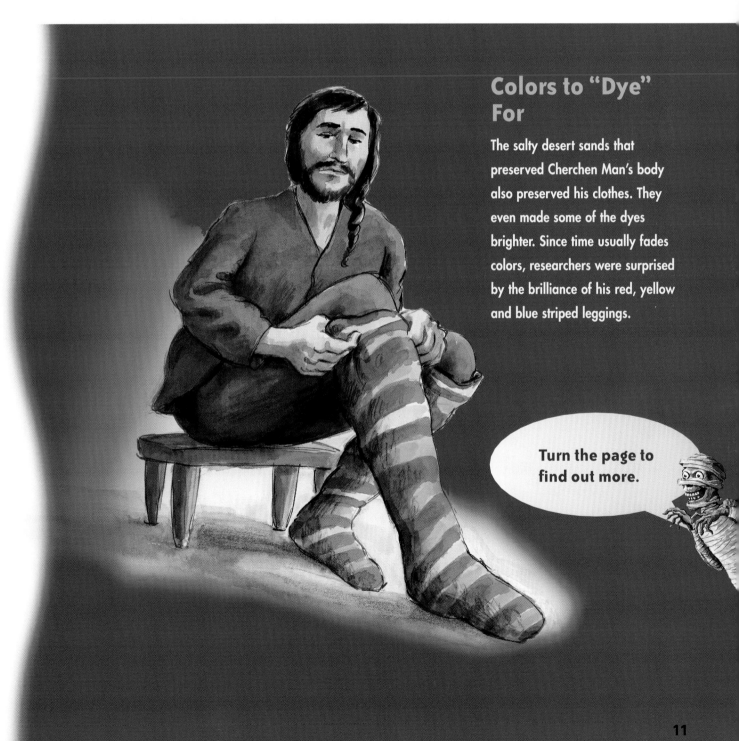

Colors to "Dye" For

The salty desert sands that preserved Cherchen Man's body also preserved his clothes. They even made some of the dyes brighter. Since time usually fades colors, researchers were surprised by the brilliance of his red, yellow and blue striped leggings.

Turn the page to find out more.

11

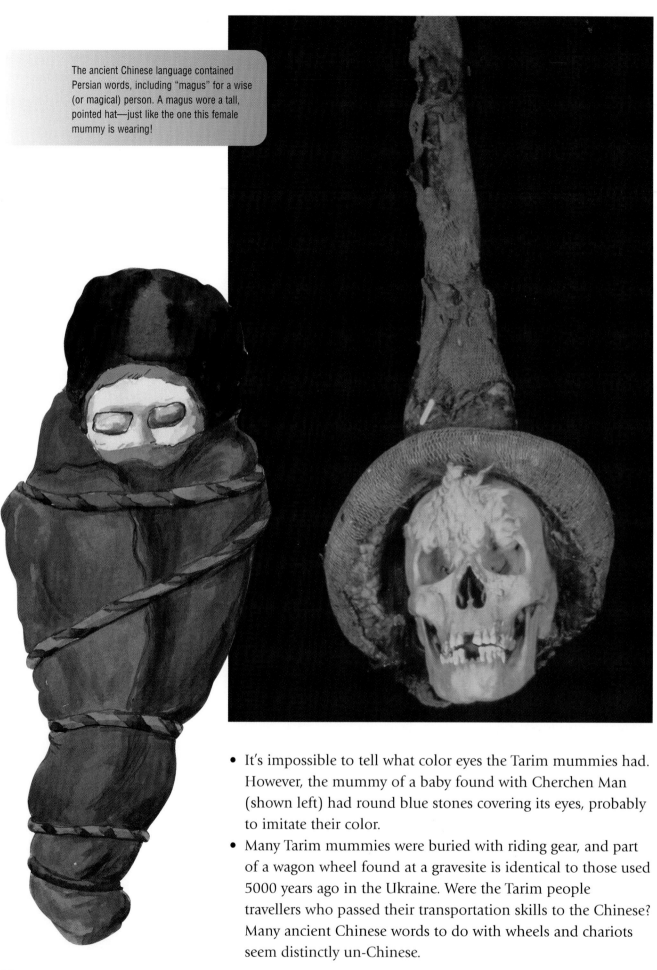

- It's impossible to tell what color eyes the Tarim mummies had. However, the mummy of a baby found with Cherchen Man (shown left) had round blue stones covering its eyes, probably to imitate their color.
- Many Tarim mummies were buried with riding gear, and part of a wagon wheel found at a gravesite is identical to those used 5000 years ago in the Ukraine. Were the Tarim people travellers who passed their transportation skills to the Chinese? Many ancient Chinese words to do with wheels and chariots seem distinctly un-Chinese.

- Ancient manuscripts found in the Tarim Basin were in a language called Tokharian, which is similar to Celtic languages. The Celts—tall blond people with blue-gray eyes—spread west from central Europe 2400 years ago. Could the Tokharians have been Celts who headed east two thousand years early? No one knows, but the Tarim mummies look like Tokharians shown in pictures, and fair-haired blue-eyed people still live in the Tarim Basin.

- Some of the mummies at the northern end of the Tarim Basin were dressed or wrapped (see right) in cloth that was tartan, a kind of plaid made on a special European loom. The Tarim tartan is almost identical to tartans made by ancient Celtic tribes in Germany, Austria and Scandinavia.

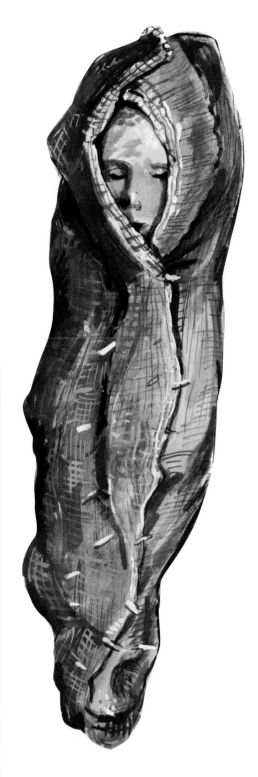

Fuzz Buzz

The oldest Tarim mummies were preserved naturally. But nature might have had a helping hand with some of the younger mummies, including Cherchen Man. Their skin was covered with a strange yellow fuzz. The fuzz is definitely animal protein, but what kind remains a mystery. It has the look of 5000-year-old whipped egg whites. Many mummies found in the Andean mountains of Peru were also painted with animal protein. But in their case, it was fish paste. A smelly insect repellent?

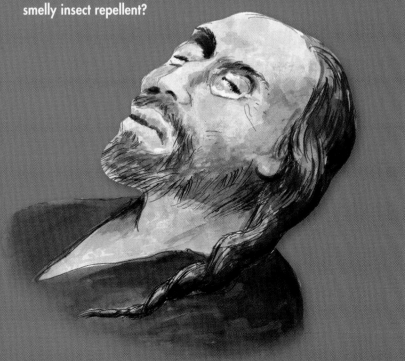

BOG
Bodies

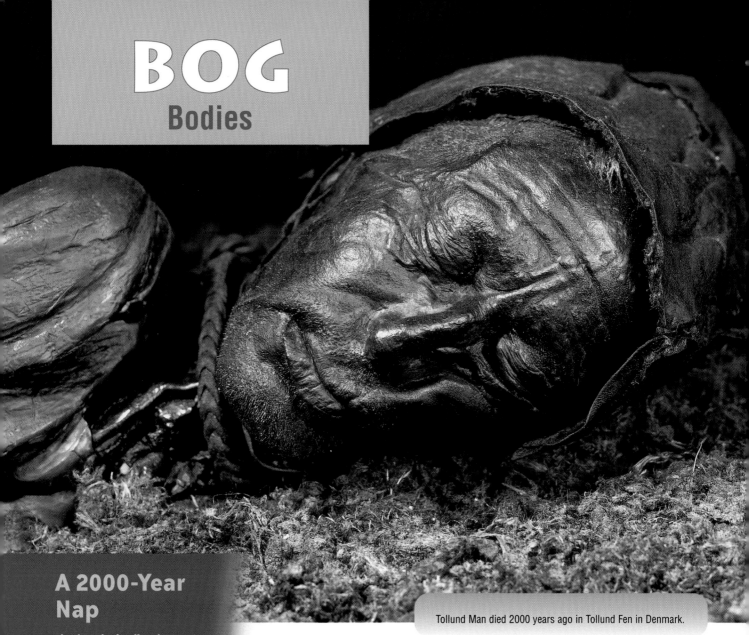

Tollund Man died 2000 years ago in Tollund Fen in Denmark.

A 2000-Year Nap

The head of Tollund Man (see above) is particularly well preserved. His peaceful facial expression makes it look as if he just might be enjoying an afternoon nap. But if you look a little more carefully, you can see a braided rope around his neck. Does that mean he met his death by hanging or, as others believe, could the rope be a kind of religious symbol?

On May 8, 1950, two men were working in a bog, or swamp, in Denmark. They were digging out peat, partially decomposed plant matter, to use as fuel. Imagine their surprise when they found a human face sticking out of the bog! They uncovered a man's body, preserved in the peat, with a rope around its neck. What they thought was a recent murder victim turned out to be a preserved body that had been lying in the bog since the Iron Age (the centuries where BC meets AD).

Tollund Man is only one of many bodies found in the peat bogs of northern Europe. Peat bogs preserve bodies extremely well. The peat in the bog cuts off the oxygen that bacteria need to survive. Acidic water quickly soaks into a body, preserving everything, even the bits inside that usually rot first. But it softens bones until they become spongy, so many bog bodies end up being squashed flat.

It's understandable that Tollund Man was mistaken for a murder victim. Some bog bodies are so well preserved they seem to have spent only a short time buried. And many bodies from the Iron Age had violent deaths. When two Englishmen found the head of a woman in Lindow Moss, a bog in Cheshire, a local man thought they had found his missing wife—and confessed to her murder! (The bog woman actually had died 1700 years earlier.) A "stick" found in the same bog turned out to be the leg of 2000-year-old Lindow Man, who had been struck from behind and strangled with a cord, and then had his throat slit. Were these people executed or maybe sacrificed to an Iron Age god?

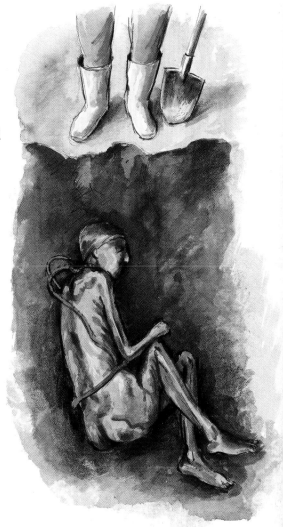

Soggy Sacrifices?

- The contents of many bog people's stomachs show they died in winter or early spring.
  Explanation? Roman writers describe Iron Age mid-winter and spring festivals during which people were sacrificed in watery bogs.
- Many bog bodies have twisted ropes around their necks.
  Explanation? They might be religious symbols. They look similar to the twisted neck-rings that were the mark of the Earth Mother goddess.
- Many bog people have well-manicured fingernails.
  Explanation? They might have been attendants to the goddess. In return for an easy life, some were sacrificed.
- Lindow Man's stomach contained burnt bread.
  Explanation? During the spring festival of Beltain, special bread was broken up and handed around. Whoever received the burnt portion was sacrificed to ensure a good harvest.

Putting a Face to the Name

Just as forensic scientists use remains of victims to solve murders, forensic anthropologists and artists worked from measurements of Lindow Man's skull to come up with a face for him (right). His skeleton tells us he was 1.68 m (5 ft 6 in) tall, weighed about 60 kg (132 lb) and must have been in his twenties when he met his violent death.

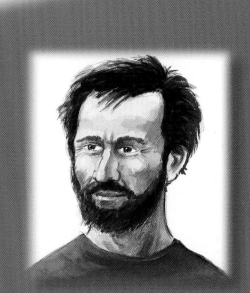

JUANITA,
the Inca Ice Maiden

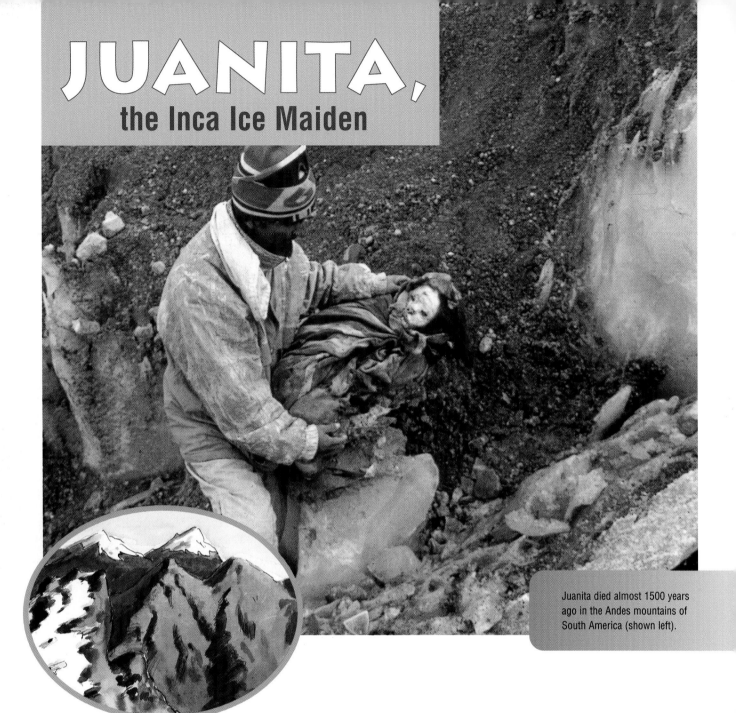

Juanita died almost 1500 years ago in the Andes mountains of South America (shown left).

The last turn of the millennium, the year AD 1000, was as eventful as the most recent one. The Vikings were in Newfoundland, the Chinese were having fun with fireworks . . . and the Inca people in South America were building their capital city of Cuczo, center of an empire that would last until the Spanish conquest 500 years later. The empire stretched from what is now Peru, all the way down the mountainous spine of South America to Argentina.

The Incas saw the peaks of the Andes mountains as powerful gods, and they offered sacrifices in return for rain and full harvests. At times of great danger, the Incas climbed to the top of their sacred mountains to be close to Inti, the Sun God, and offered him the most precious gift of all—the lives of their children.

In 1995, hot ash from a volcano melted 500 years' accumulation of ice from the summit of Mount Ampato—revealing the mummy of a beautiful 13-year-old girl, later named Juanita. Arrangements were quickly made to recover her body and take it down the mountain before it had a chance to thaw. Juanita's body had naturally dried and mummified in the freezing conditions on the mountaintop. Her face had decayed a little, but the rest of her body was so well preserved that researchers can even study her DNA.

The Chosen One

To be chosen for sacrifice was a great honor, usually bestowed on the children of Inca chiefs. By going willingly, Juanita became a god, and forever linked her family with the Inca king, who was thought to be a descendant of Inti, the Sun God.

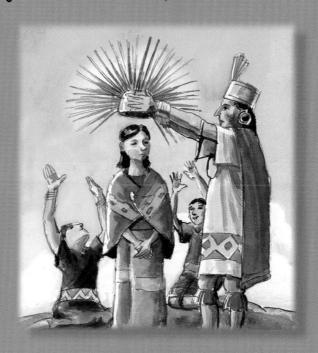

Day of the Living Dead

Every year in mid-winter, the Inca people celebrated the Festival of Inti. The Inca king led the Procession of the Living Dead to the Temple of the Sun. Former Inca kings, wearing beautiful capes and golden masks, were carried through the crowds. They sat cross-legged on litters balanced on men's shoulders—not a heavy load, as the kings were mummies whose bodies had dried out in the high mountains. These mummy kings were housed in great palaces, and offered the best food and drink. They acted as messengers between Inti and the Inca people, and ensured that Inti rose high in the sky every year so that summer would return to the land.

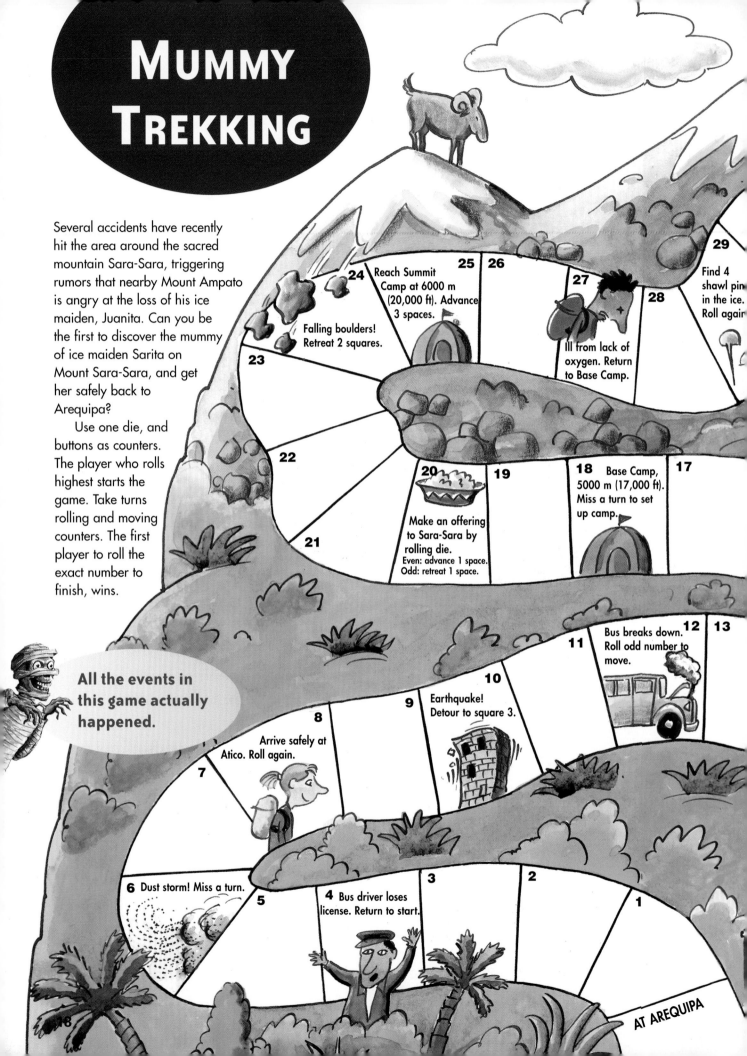

MUMMY TREKKING

Several accidents have recently hit the area around the sacred mountain Sara-Sara, triggering rumors that nearby Mount Ampato is angry at the loss of his ice maiden, Juanita. Can you be the first to discover the mummy of ice maiden Sarita on Mount Sara-Sara, and get her safely back to Arequipa?

Use one die, and buttons as counters. The player who rolls highest starts the game. Take turns rolling and moving counters. The first player to roll the exact number to finish, wins.

All the events in this game actually happened.

24 Falling boulders! Retreat 2 squares.

23

22

21

25 26

25 Reach Summit Camp at 6000 m (20,000 ft). Advance 3 spaces.

20 Make an offering to Sara-Sara by rolling die. Even: advance 1 space. Odd: retreat 1 space.

19

27 Ill from lack of oxygen. Return to Base Camp.

28

29 Find 4 shawl pin in the ice. Roll agair

18 Base Camp, 5000 m (17,000 ft). Miss a turn to set up camp.

17

11

12 13

12 Bus breaks down. Roll odd number to move.

10 Earthquake! Detour to square 3.

9

8 Arrive safely at Atico. Roll again.

7

6 Dust storm! Miss a turn.

5

4 Bus driver loses license. Return to start.

3

2

1

AT AREQUIPA

18

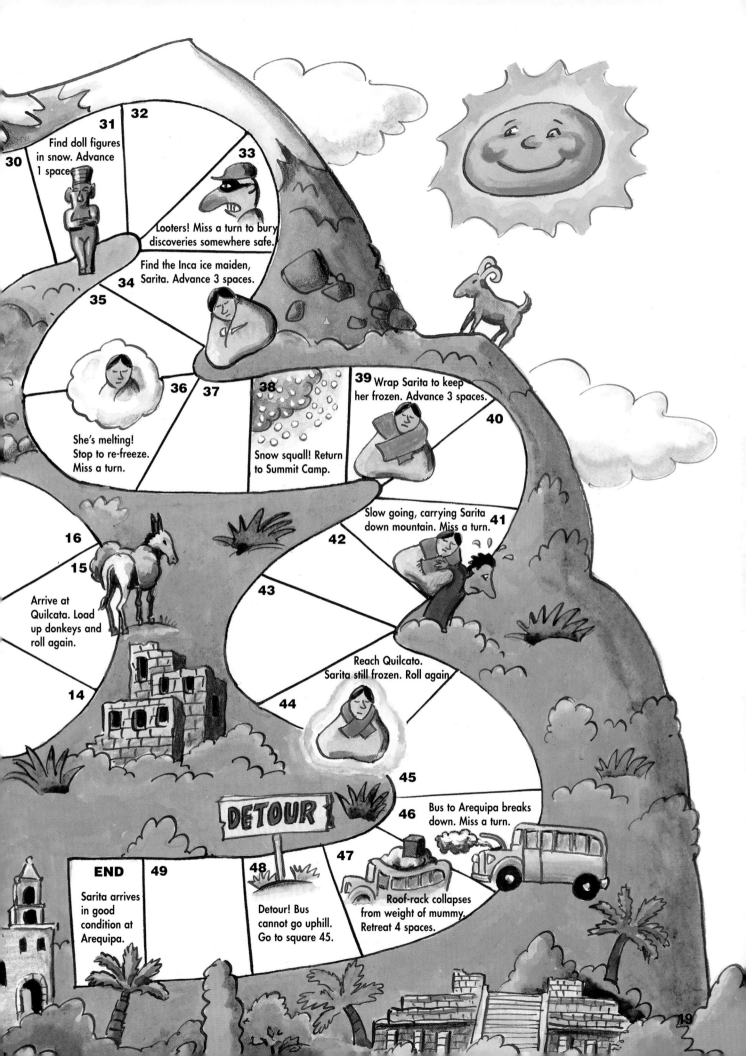

30

31 **32**
Find doll figures in snow. Advance 1 space.

33
Looters! Miss a turn to bury discoveries somewhere safe.

Find the Inca ice maiden, Sarita. Advance 3 spaces.

34

35

36 **37**
She's melting! Stop to re-freeze. Miss a turn.

38
Snow squall! Return to Summit Camp.

39 Wrap Sarita to keep her frozen. Advance 3 spaces.

40

16

15
Arrive at Quilcata. Load up donkeys and roll again.

14

Slow going, carrying Sarita down mountain. Miss a turn. **41**

42

43

Reach Quilcato. Sarita still frozen. Roll again

44

45

DETOUR

46 Bus to Arequipa breaks down. Miss a turn.

END

49

48
Detour! Bus cannot go uphill. Go to square 45.

47
Roof-rack collapses from weight of mummy. Retreat 4 spaces.

Sarita arrives in good condition at Arequipa.

SNOW Mummies

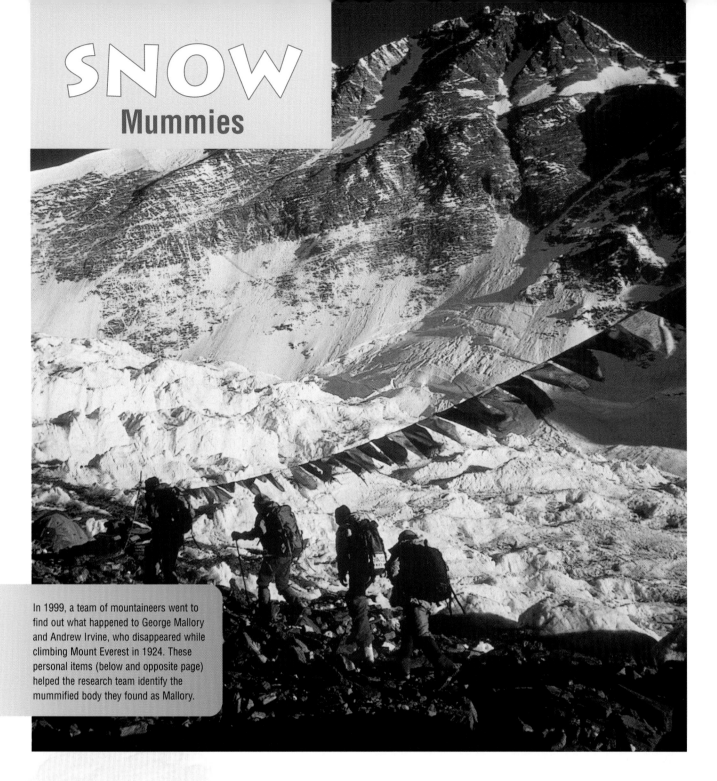

In 1999, a team of mountaineers went to find out what happened to George Mallory and Andrew Irvine, who disappeared while climbing Mount Everest in 1924. These personal items (below and opposite page) helped the research team identify the mummified body they found as Mallory.

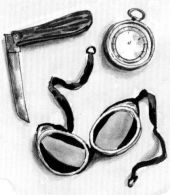

On the morning of June 8, 1924, George Mallory and Andrew Irvine set out on the last leg of their climb to the top of Mount Everest. They carried a photo of Mallory's wife to leave at the summit and a camera to take pictures there. But they never returned. Seventy-five years later, members of the Mallory and Irvine Research Expedition set out to solve the mystery of what happened to the two climbers. The big question: did the mountain take their lives before or after they conquered it?

The research team expected to find the body of Irvine, because it had been sighted in 1975. But they were unprepared for their discovery 600 m (1970 ft) below the summit. Stretched out, fingers dug deeply into the gravel, was the mummified body of a man. There was no doubting his identity. The body looked like Mallory, the clothes bore his name tags and the pockets contained letters addressed to him.

There was no photo, and the camera was missing. Did the climbers reach the summit, leave the photo there and record their conquest on film? With luck, the camera will be found with Irvine's body, the film as well preserved as Mallory's body in the frigid conditions at the top of the world.

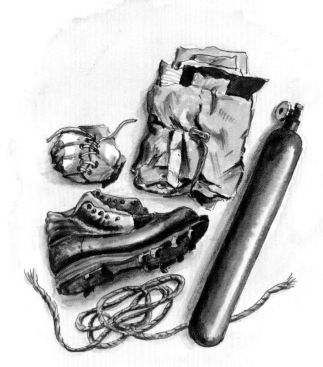

A-Hunting We Will Go

Three teachers were hunting for dall sheep in the northern British Columbia homeland of the Champagne and Aishihik First Nations (CAFN), when they met another hunter. But this one lived more than 300 years before European people reached the northwest coast. The mummified body of a man—carrying hunting gear (right)—was revealed as the glacier that preserved it for 550 years melted. The CAFN elders named him Kwaday Dan Sinchi, which means "long-ago person found."

The Face of an Explorer

The body of John Torrington was found on Beechey Island in the Canadian Arctic in 1984. Torrington, a member of the doomed Franklin Expedition to find the Northwest Passage, died in the winter of 1845. Yet when his coffin was opened, the scientists found a perfectly preserved body. The possible cause of Torrington's death was also preserved—a pile of empty food tins sealed with melted tin and lead. The expedition's vast store of preserved food—containing lethal dissolved lead—turned out to be more dangerous than marauding polar bears or the iron grip of an Arctic winter.

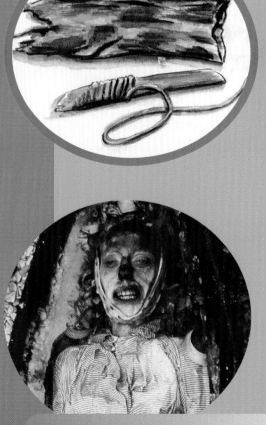

Explorer John Torrington died in 1845.

ANIMALS
Have Mummies, Too

The Bluest Mummy

Who was Blue Babe? He was an eight-year-old bison who was killed one winter by a lion. As he froze and became part of the permafrost near Fairbanks, Alaska, for the next 36,000 years, a chemical reaction turned him blue! We know that Blue Babe's killer was a type of lion, from the size of the scratches and bites on his body, and because a piece of tooth embedded in his skin had the thick enamel found on a lion's teeth. The annual growth rings in Blue Babe's own teeth and horns gave away his age—one ring for each year of life. And because Blue Babe had lots of underfur in his coat and a thick layer of fat under his skin, we know he died during cold weather.

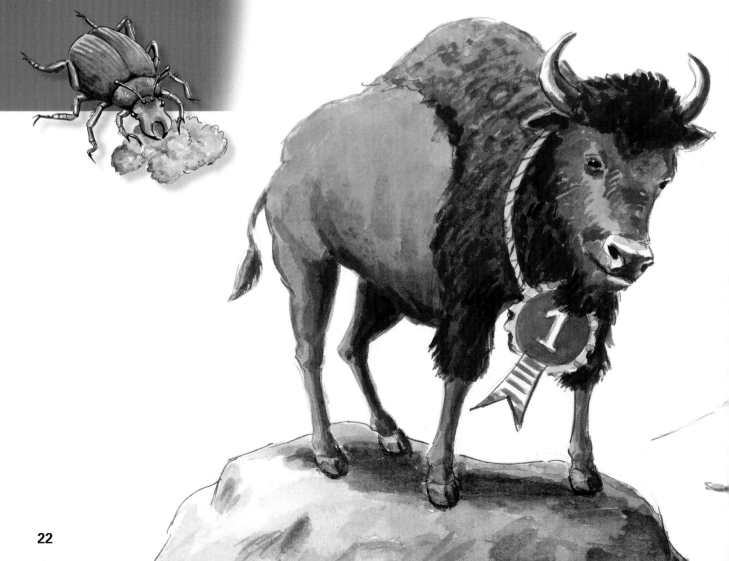

The Oldest Mummy

In the movie Jurassic Park, scientists used a blood cell found inside a blood-sucking insect—trapped in a piece of amber—to clone a dinosaur. Forget about whether they could actually do that, and concentrate on the amber. Amber is fossilized resin, the sticky stuff that oozes out of trees. Besides forming an airtight seal around a body, resin destroys body-rotting bacteria and fungi. The oldest mummy ever found was an insect trapped inside a piece of fossilized resin 310 million years old! The resin had hardened, but the insect had been preserved exactly as it was when it died (right).

The Biggest Mummy

In 1900 a Siberian hunter came upon what he thought was a gigantic mole that had burrowed up through the ground and died. His huge mole turned out to be a mammoth, whose frozen body had surfaced as the icy ground melted around it. One of the most perfectly preserved mammoths found in the Siberian tundra was a six-month-old baby mammoth, later named Dima. He died 40,000 years ago and caused a big stir in scientific circles when he was discovered in 1977, because he was the first complete mammoth that scientists had had a chance to study.

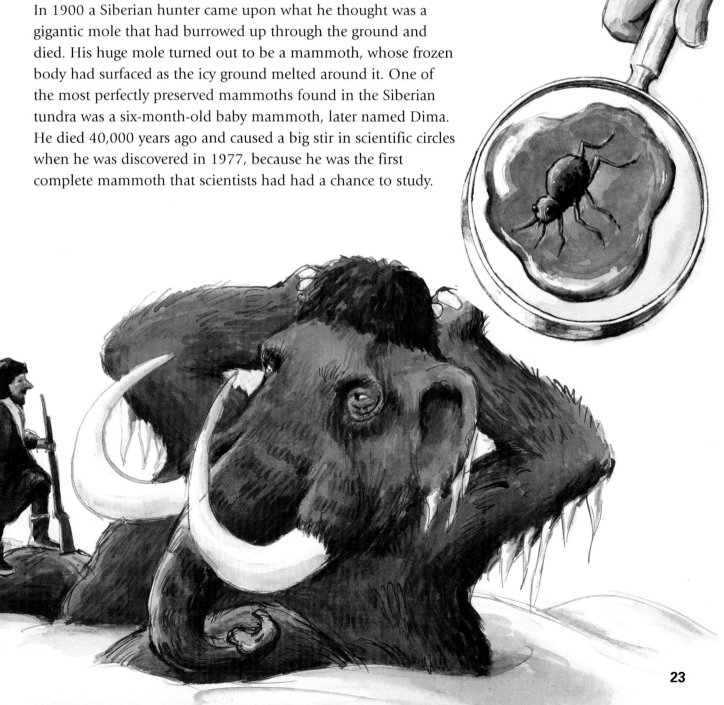

The CHINCHORRO Mummies

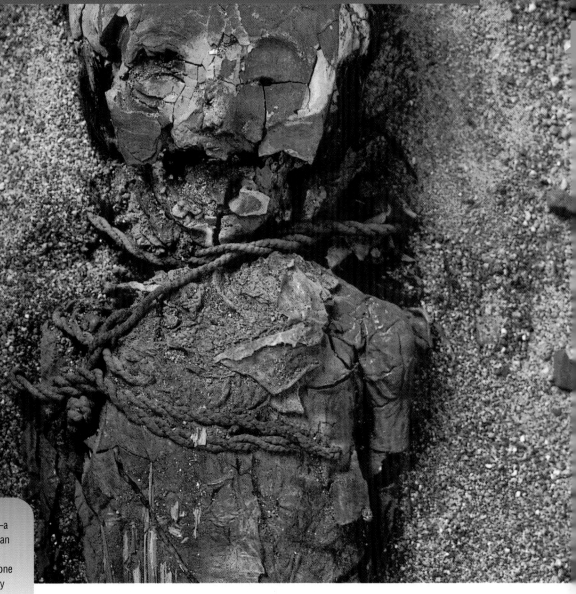

This black-painted mummy—a young boy who died more than 7000 years ago on the west coast of South America—is one of the oldest known artificially created mummies.

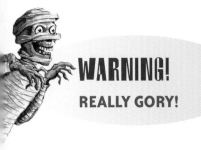

WARNING!
REALLY GORY!

A long the coastline of northern Chile, a few mountain streams manage to cross the dry Atacama Desert and form green valleys at the coast. Groups of prehistoric hunter-gatherers, people we call the Chinchorro, lived here. They found plenty of food in the Pacific Ocean, and when food is easy to find, people have time for other things—like developing religious beliefs and creating mummies to act as links between the living and the dead. The Chinchorro people did exactly that, more than 2000 years before the idea caught on in ancient Egypt.

Beneath the black paint of a Chinchorro mummy is a body that has been taken apart and put back together again. The process begins with the removal of the dead person's head, arms and legs. The body skin is carefully rolled back and stored in a jar of seawater to keep it supple. After the internal organs and brain are taken out, the inside of the body is dried with hot coals. Then the arm bones and leg bones are removed and cleaned.

To reassemble the body, the mummy-maker builds a stick frame, lashes it to the bones, and runs it through the chest up into the head. Next, the chest cavity is stuffed with grass and ash, and the body padded with reeds. A thick paste made from white ash is spread all over the body. Then comes the tricky part, pulling the skin back over the body—if it doesn't fit, it is patched with animal skin. A wig is glued to the head and the hands and feet are attached with reed cord. All that's left to do now is paint the mummy black and buff the dried paint with a smooth pebble.

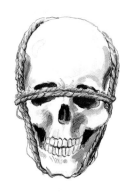

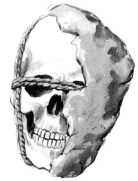

Once the skull was cleaned, it was tied together with reed cords. The face was re-built using a paste made from ashes. After the skin and hair was put back on the skull, the mask was covered with a mineral paint.

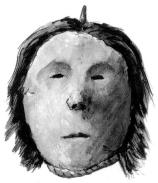

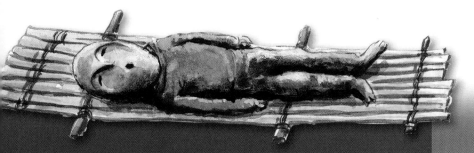

Anyone Can Apply

Mummification, connecting the world of the living with that of the dead, was a religious act for the Chinchorro people. Unlike the early Egyptians, who thought that only kings and other important people deserved an afterlife, the Chinchorro mummified anyone who died. This baby (above) was buried with the stick frame that would have been its cradleboard while it was alive. Newborns, and even unborn fetuses, were lovingly preserved.

Mummies Made Simple

After about 3000 BC, Chinchorro mummy-makers stopped making elaborate black mummies. They began to simply remove the soft bits from inside a body, stuff it with earth, cover it with paste and paint it red. Later, they made their job even easier by leaving the body intact and coating it with a thick layer of mud.

It's a WRAP!

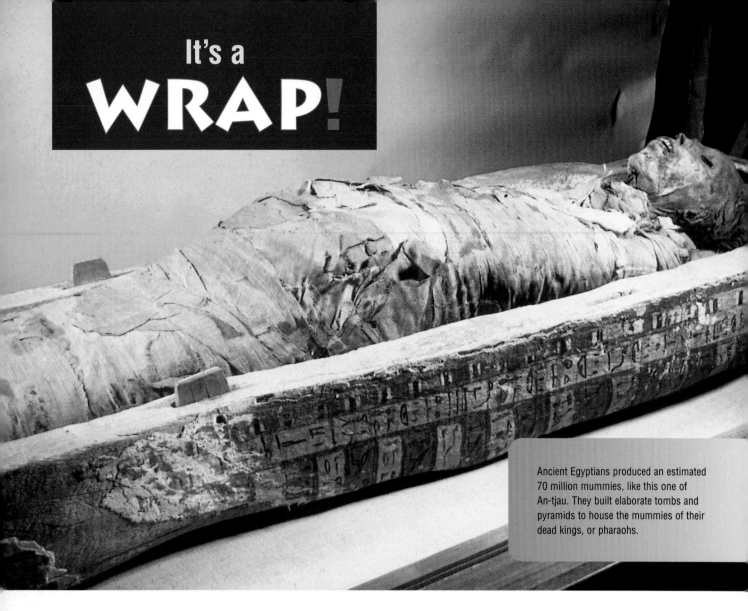

Ancient Egyptians produced an estimated 70 million mummies, like this one of An-tjau. They built elaborate tombs and pyramids to house the mummies of their dead kings, or pharaohs.

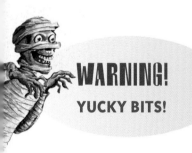

WARNING!
YUCKY BITS!

Before 3100 BC, tribes along the River Nile buried their dead in pits in the desert. The dry sand sucked out all the moisture to make the oldest, best-preserved mummies found in the Nile valley, without a single bandage! After the tribes united to form Egypt, they buried pharaohs (their kings) in coffins and tombs. Big mistake! Deprived of contact with the sand, these bodies rotted away. So the Egyptians experimented with preserving dead bodies for the next 3000 years.

From the Early Period (up to 2650 BC)—when bodies were dried with natron salt, wrapped in resin-soaked bandages and buried curled up on their sides—to the time when mummy-making became a fine art (1070–712 BC), mummies changed as Egyptian religious beliefs changed. At first only pharaohs, who were thought to be living gods, were mummified. Then, the idea got around that everyone's spirit could make the trip to the land of the gods, and the mummy business took off.

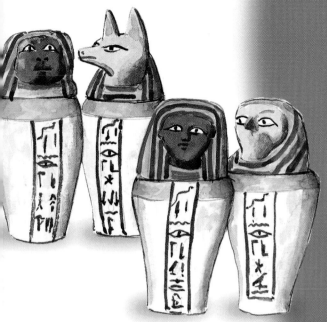

Ka

Each time the ram-headed god Khnum makes a human baby out of clay, he also makes a spirit double—or ka. After death the ka remains with the body, and the food in the tomb is for the ka, not the mummy.

Ba

The ba, or personality of the dead person, is shown as a human-headed bird. During the funeral, a priest touches the mummy with a special instrument, which releases the ba from the body. It flies to the burial chamber and perches close to the body.

Akh

Mummy-makers recite prayers and magical spells to create the akh, the spiritual part of the dead person. Using the mummified body as a vehicle, the akh journeys through the underworld and finds the entrance to the afterlife.

Heart

To be accepted among the gods, the dead person must deny bad deeds in front of the god Osiris. Then his or her heart is weighed against the feather of truth (below). If the scales tip, the heart is eaten by the Devourer of the Dead—no afterlife for this mummy!

Mummies became more lifelike. The body was laid flat so the mummy-maker could reach inside to remove the body organs, which were housed in canopic jars (above). Special tools were used to remove the brain through the nose. Padding under the skin looked good, except when well-packed mummies burst as their skin shrank!

As the Egyptian kingdom started to decline, mummy-makers took less care with their work. They tried out fancy bandaging to cover poorly preserved bodies. The bodies were pumped full of resin, creating the sticky "black pitch" bodies that the Arabs later named *moumia*, which gave us our word "mummy."

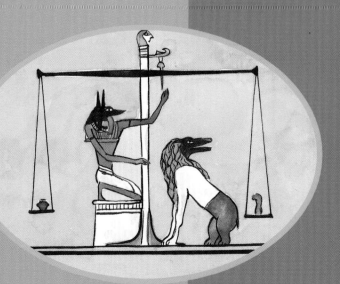

MAKE A MINI-MUMMY

How does nature make a mummy? Find out for yourself.

You'll need:
- A small, fresh apple (Golden Delicious works best)
- A sharp knife (ask permission)
- A small bowl
- Lemon juice
- Paper towel
- A wire coat hanger
- 2 whole cloves
- Pipe cleaners
- Cloth material (old rags)

Step 1

Peel the apple and make small cuts in it like this:
- two wrinkles on forehead
- two small holes for eyes
- one deep cut down each side of nose
- three cuts to form the mouth and chin (like this)

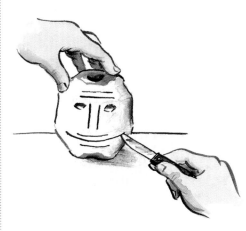

Soak the apple thoroughly for 10 seconds in lemon juice, making sure the juice gets into all the cuts.

Step 2

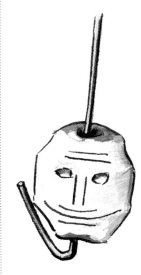

Straighten the coat hanger. Push it right through the apple core. Bend both ends of the hanger into hooks. Hang up the apple some-place dry. (Not the kitchen or bathroom.)

Step 3

After two weeks, remove the coat hanger and mold the apple into a mummy head. Gently push in the lower part of the cheeks, pull down the chin and shape the nose. Push a clove into each eye hole. Hang up the head on its hanger to continue mummifying.

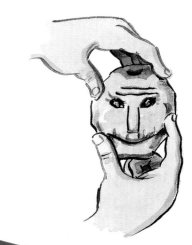

Mummy Muffins

Remember the natural salt—natron—that the ancient Egyptians packed their mummies in to dry them out? It contains large amounts of sodium bicarbonate. You might know it as baking soda. Yes, that's right—mummy salt helps make delicious cakes!

Step 4

After two more weeks, shape a body out of pipe cleaners, giving it a neck long enough to skewer the mummy head.

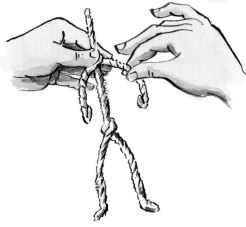

Step 5

Bandage the arms and legs with strips of old material, pad out the chest with more material and fold the arms over it.

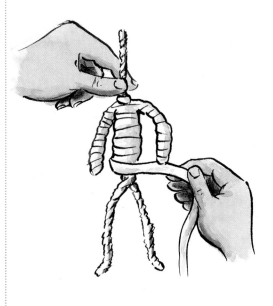

Step 6

Wrap a figure-eight bandage around the top of the head and body to hold the head in place then wrap the entire body mummy-style. Leave the face unbandaged. Write the name of your mummy on the bandages. If you know any magic words, write these too.

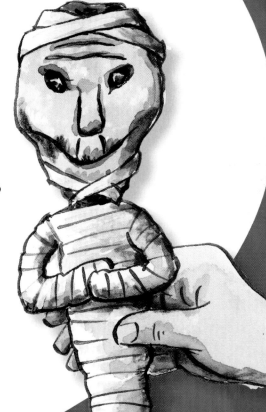

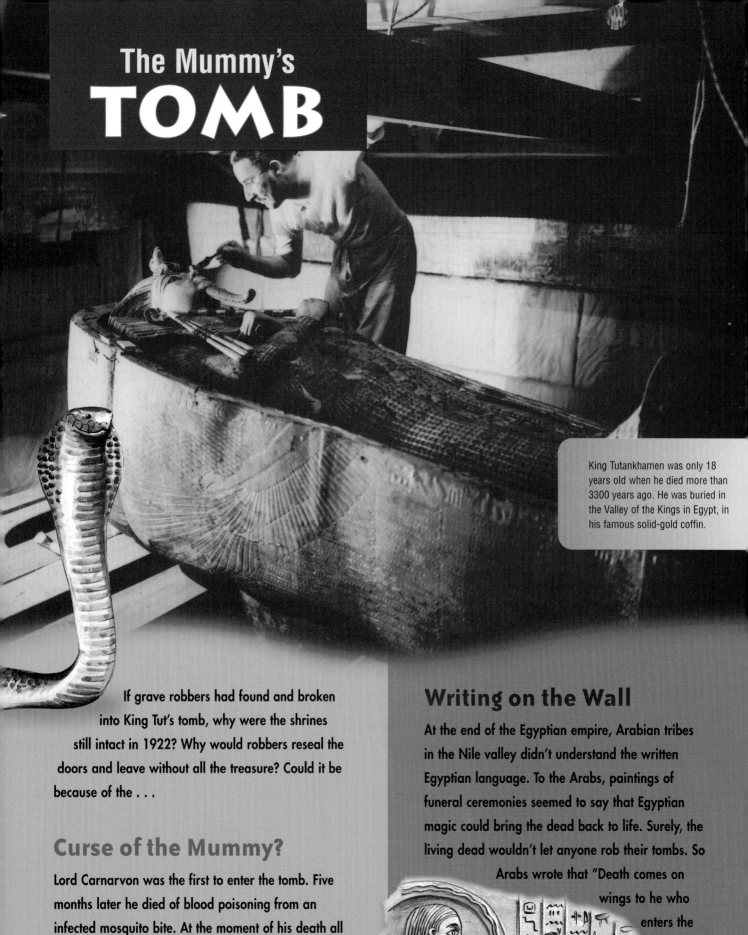

The Mummy's
TOMB

King Tutankhamen was only 18 years old when he died more than 3300 years ago. He was buried in the Valley of the Kings in Egypt, in his famous solid-gold coffin.

If grave robbers had found and broken into King Tut's tomb, why were the shrines still intact in 1922? Why would robbers reseal the doors and leave without all the treasure? Could it be because of the . . .

Curse of the Mummy?

Lord Carnarvon was the first to enter the tomb. Five months later he died of blood poisoning from an infected mosquito bite. At the moment of his death all the lights in Cairo went out, while in England his fox terrier, Susie, howled once and dropped dead.

Writing on the Wall

At the end of the Egyptian empire, Arabian tribes in the Nile valley didn't understand the written Egyptian language. To the Arabs, paintings of funeral ceremonies seemed to say that Egyptian magic could bring the dead back to life. Surely, the living dead wouldn't let anyone rob their tombs. So Arabs wrote that "Death comes on wings to he who enters the tomb of a pharaoh."

By the 20th century, most of the tombs in Egypt had been plundered by grave robbers. In 1922, after a five-year search in the Valley of the Kings, Howard Carter discovered the legendary tomb of young King Tutankhamen. Follow Carter and his financial backer, Lord Carnarvon, into the tomb. . . .

A buried staircase ends at a stone door carrying King Tutankhamen's great seal. The door was broken through and resealed 3000 years ago.

Thieves had also broken through and then resealed a second door. Carter makes a small hole in it. His candle remains lit—the air is breathable. Opening the door, Carter and Lord Carnarvon gaze upon an Antechamber full of clothes, musical instruments, food and flowers, with two statues of Tutankhamen guarding the entrance to his Burial Chamber. It too bears the mark of thieves, who obviously left in a hurry—scattered beads and a scarf containing gold rings lie on the floor.

With relief, Carter realizes that the chamber's greatest treasures are intact—an immense gold shrine containing three inner shrines. Inside the last one stands a stone sarcophagus protecting three mummy-shaped coffins, nestling inside each other. The solid gold innermost coffin contains the king, and his mummy wears a solid gold mask. Surrounding the canopic chest containing the king's internal organs are statues of gods and goddesses, chariots, caskets of jewels, ostrich fans and a fleet of model boats with sails.

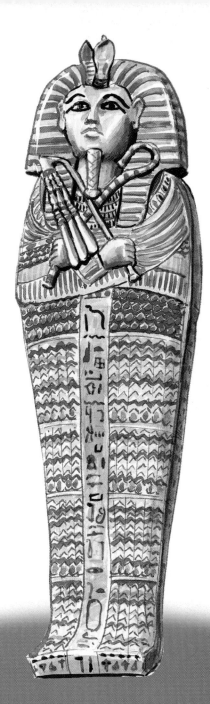

King Tut's Killer Bug

Sir Arthur Conan Doyle, the writer who created Sherlock Holmes, thought Carnarvon might have died from a deadly germ placed in the tomb. Research shows that if harmful germs had been sealed in the tomb, they would be lethal by 1922. Everything in the tomb was covered in a mysterious pink dust, and there were patches of black fungus on the walls.

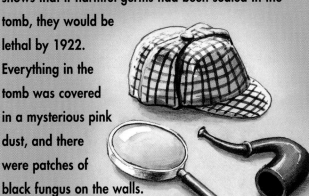

Mischievous Mummy?

In 1992, a BBC TV crew shot footage of Tutankhamen's treasures in Cairo Museum, only to find that the tape was blank when they played it back. While filming in the tomb, someone recalled the mummy's curse. Instantly, the lights went out and that person suddenly developed breathing difficulties. Later, the hotel elevator he was in plummeted 21 floors when its cable snapped!

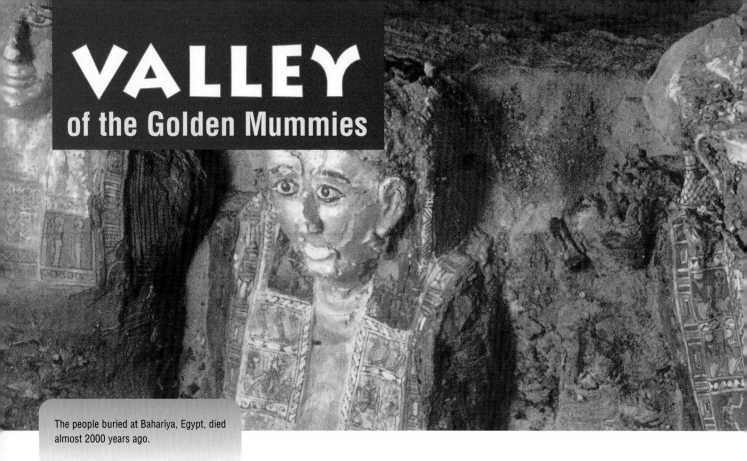

VALLEY
of the Golden Mummies

The people buried at Bahariya, Egypt, died almost 2000 years ago.

King Tut's Peas

If you're invited to lunch at the Duke of Sutherland's home in Scotland, take a helping of his delicious peas. Rumor has it that the peas growing in his garden were taken from King Tut's tomb. If the thought of eating 3000-year-old peas makes you want to gag—relax. The Duke doesn't serve the dried up peas from a moldy tomb—just peas from plants that grew from them.

The most exciting mummy discovery since the tomb of Tutankhamen occurred in 1996 in Egypt's Western Desert. A donkey accidentally put its foot through the roof of a tomb buried beneath the sand. For three years archeologists secretly excavated the site. Finally, they announced that the Bahariya oasis, southwest of Cairo, was the site of an immense ancient cemetery. It might contain as many as 10,000 mummies—and it has never been looted! The excavations at Bahariya will continue for 10 more years.

The cemetery is the resting place of wealthy families from the 1st and 2nd centuries AD, when Bahariya was a rich wine-producing region under Roman rule. The realistic portraits of the dead on their burial masks show that these Egyptians lived a Roman lifestyle. Yet they were buried in the ancient Egyptian tradition, and their tombs contain pictures of all the same gods found in Tutankhamen's tomb.

Embalmers used so much resin to preserve the mummies that its smell is still strong in the air. They wrapped some mummies in linen bandages, often forming intricate diamond patterns. They laid others to rest in terra cotta coffins shaped like human bodies. They covered others from head to waist in decorated pasteboard masks made from linen or papyrus, known as a cartonnage. They also gave many mummies exquisite golden masks topped with crowns, and often covered mummies of children in a fine layer of gold.

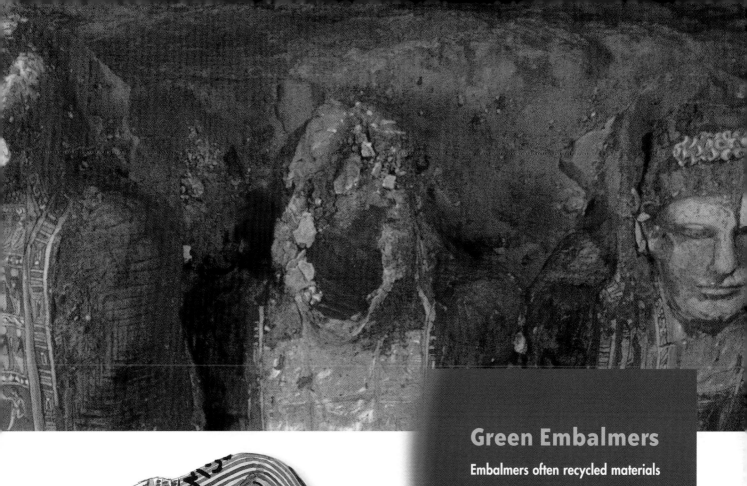

Green Embalmers

Embalmers often recycled materials when they mummified people. What if the papyrus—a kind of Egyptian paper—used to wrap some of the mummies at Bahariya was recycled? Imagine how much information these mummies could give about life 2000 years ago if the embalmers used paper with writing on it!

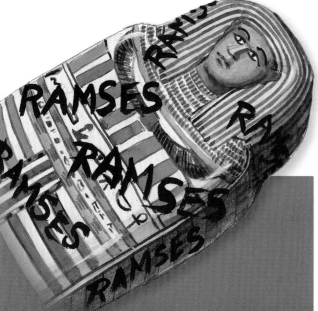

It's All in a Name

The ancient Egyptians believed that as long as a person's name was being spoken, his or her immortality was assured. That's why pharaohs' names were written all over their tombs, coffins, even mummy wrappings. The greatest horror to all Egyptians was to have their names removed from their tombs.

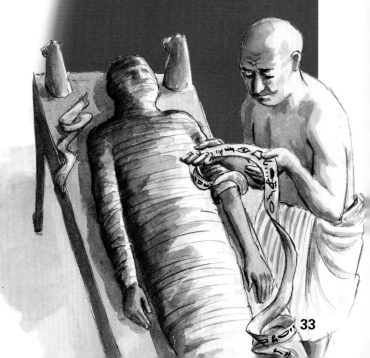

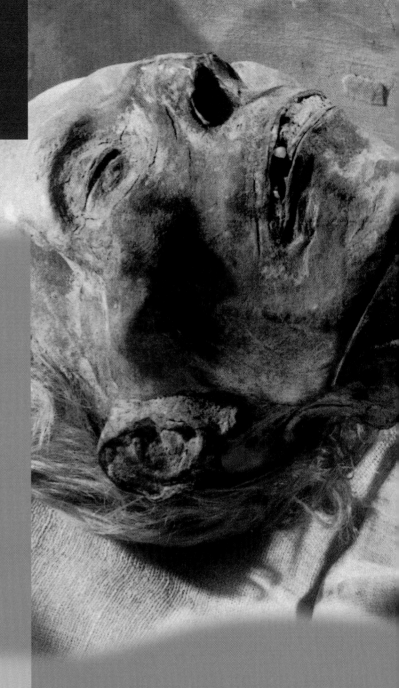

ASK
a Mummy

What's the Scariest Thing a Mummy Has Ever Done?

In 1881, when Egyptian authorities clamped down on the illegal activities of a notorious family of grave robbers, they discovered the family had made a fabulous find—a secret royal burial chamber. It took days to raise all the coffins, and the mummy of King Ramses II was left out in the heat and sun for so long that the resins in his wrappings began to melt. Suddenly, all work ceased and workmen stared, their eyes round with fear, as the mummy's arm slowly rose into the air!

Do Mummies Smell?

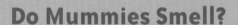

Most mummies, especially those preserved with resin and herbs, have a sort of sweet smell. However, once in a while a mummy turns up that really stinks. One found in Cairo in 1886 was wrapped in a sheepskin in a wooden coffin. When the sheepskin was cut open, everyone ran for fresh air. The dry tomb and the airtight sheepskin had preserved the body, but not fast enough to prevent some decay.

Are Mummies Still Being Made?

If you'd like to be mummified after you die, call a company in Salt Lake City. They'll dip you in a secret sauce, cover you with plastic, bind you up with linen bandages, coat you in resin and seal you in a mummy-shaped coffin of stainless steel or bronze. You have three choices of coffin, with or without hieroglyphics telling the story of your life. And you can display your coffin anywhere, as long as it doesn't block the traffic.

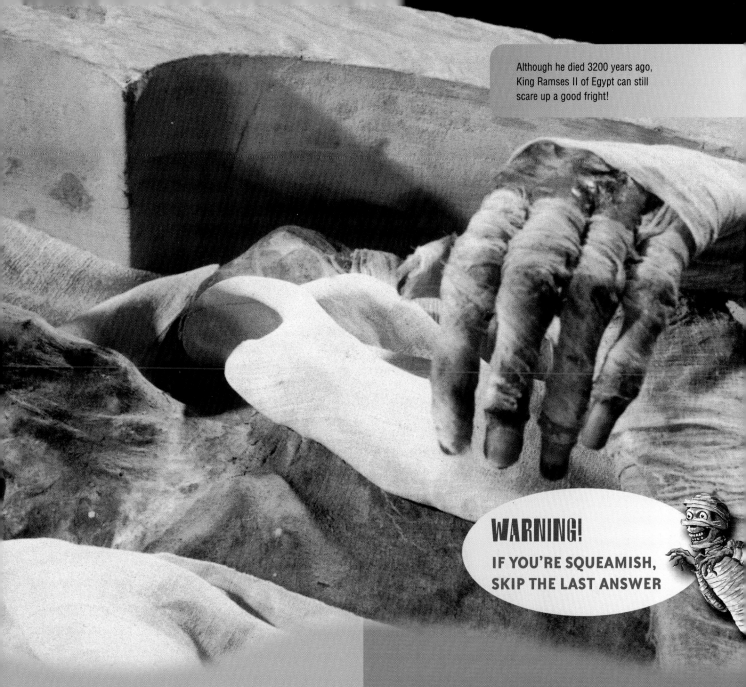

Although he died 3200 years ago, King Ramses II of Egypt can still scare up a good fright!

WARNING!
IF YOU'RE SQUEAMISH, SKIP THE LAST ANSWER

Do Mummies Fly First Class When They Travel?

No, because airline passengers have a thing about sitting next to a dead person. Mummies always travel in coffins, so they have to go in the cargo hold. And they must travel with a passport. When the mummy of Ramses II flew from Cairo to Paris for treatment of a skin condition, his passport listed his occupation as King (deceased). This entitled him to a guard of honor and a ceremonial salute at the airport.

What's a Mummy Potion?

If you went to a "doctor" in the Middle Ages and asked for something to rub on a bruise, you might have been handed an expensive jar of mummy potion—made from the melted oils from a boiled mummy. Just be glad you didn't complain of an upset stomach. The treatment for that was a dose of mummy powder—made from ground-up mummy.

Mummies Telling
TALES

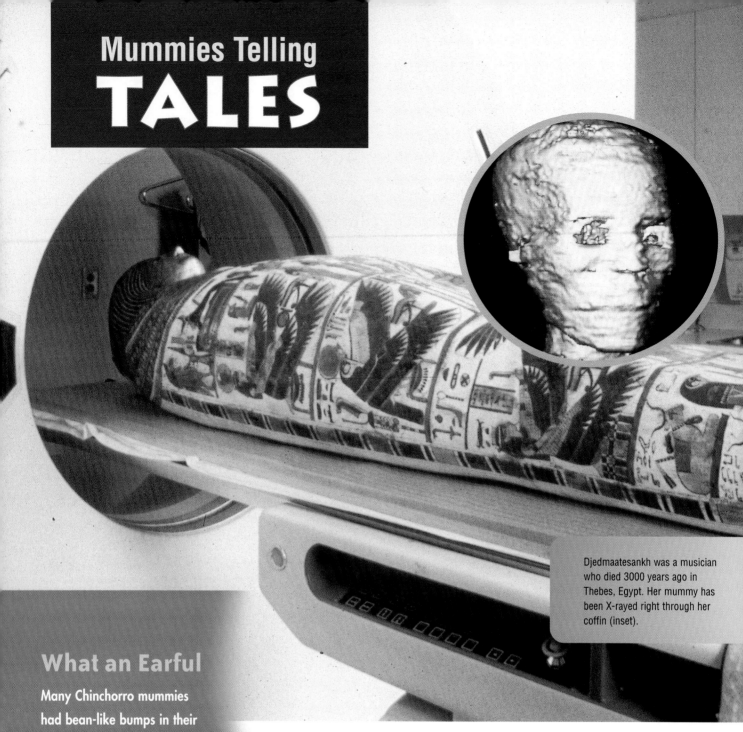

Djedmaatesankh was a musician who died 3000 years ago in Thebes, Egypt. Her mummy has been X-rayed right through her coffin (inset).

What an Earful

Many Chinchorro mummies had bean-like bumps in their ear canals caused by repeated exposure to cold water. This tells us that these people used to dive to collect shellfish. We know that most of their food came from the sea, because their teeth were worn down from the sand in their food.

Mummies have lots of stories to tell of times gone by. To discover their secrets, scientists used to unwrap them and cut them open—but that's no longer necessary. Recently, an unusual patient named Djedmaatesankh was taken from the Royal Ontario Museum to a Toronto hospital. She was once a musician in a temple in Karnak, Egypt. Now she's a mummy. Djedmaatesankh was X-rayed by a CAT-scan machine—sealed coffin and all. The scanner took hundreds of picture "slices" through the coffin, her bandages and her body. Then a computer stacked the pictures together to make a 3-D image of her.

For the first time in 3000 years, people saw what Djedmaatesankh looked like, inside and out. Scientists could tell from her bones and the wear on her teeth that she was no more than 35 years old when she died. The shape of her pelvic bones told them she'd never had children. And a 3-D picture inside her skull showed the probable cause of death—an awful tooth abscess in her jaw, which burst and spread the infection throughout her body.

Today, scientists can find out about mummies by testing their blood, analyzing their DNA and looking into their bodies through tubes called endoscopes. As new technology develops, we'll be able to find out answers to questions about mummies that we haven't even thought up yet. What we know already, however, is that when mummies were living people, they suffered from the same ailments that people do now. They had the same kinds of concerns about life and death. If you could travel back in time and talk to them, you might find you have a lot in common.

Columbus in the Clear

European settlers have finally been cleared of introducing infectious tuberculosis to South America. Fragments of DNA from tuberculosis bacteria have been found in a 1000-year-old Peruvian mummy. Since there were no European settlers in South America that long ago, the disease must already have been there when they arrived.

The Rebel Pharaoh

When Akhenaten became pharaoh of Egypt, he threw out all the old gods and insisted that everyone worship Aten, the Sun God. The reason for Akhenaten's rebellious nature was a mystery, until a Canadian student was struck by how similar he looked to present-day sufferers of a rare disorder called Marfan's Syndrome. People with this disease are tall and thin, with long, thin faces and spidery fingers. They feel isolated from others and often feel the need to rebel.

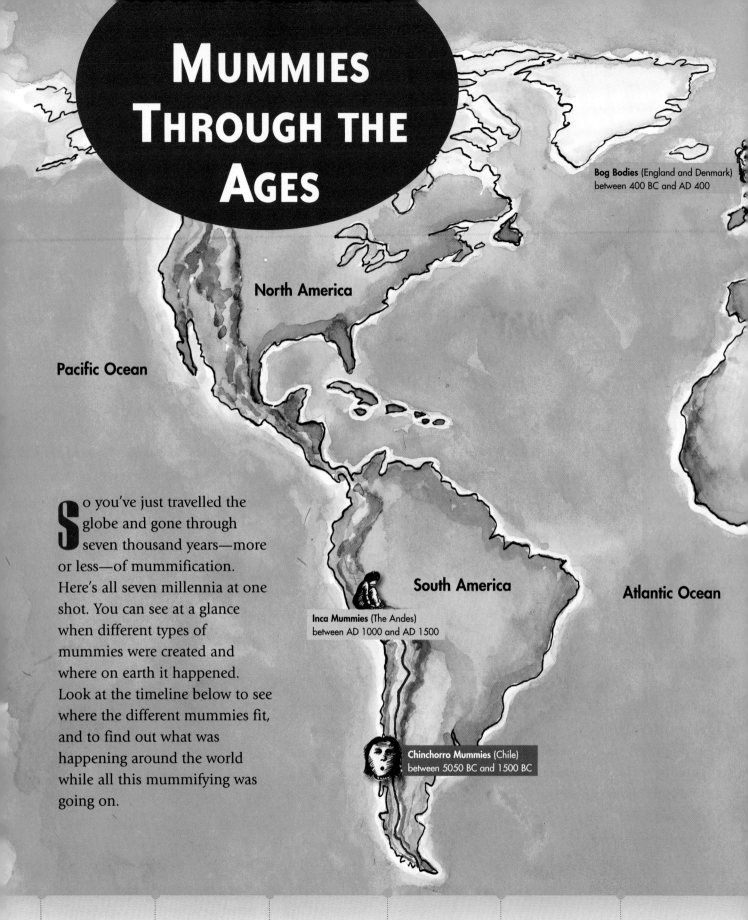

MUMMIES THROUGH THE AGES

Bog Bodies (England and Denmark) between 400 BC and AD 400

North America

Pacific Ocean

So you've just travelled the globe and gone through seven thousand years—more or less—of mummification. Here's all seven millennia at one shot. You can see at a glance when different types of mummies were created and where on earth it happened. Look at the timeline below to see where the different mummies fit, and to find out what was happening around the world while all this mummifying was going on.

South America

Atlantic Ocean

Inca Mummies (The Andes) between AD 1000 and AD 1500

Chinchorro Mummies (Chile) between 5050 BC and 1500 BC

10,000 BC
Farming is invented in the Near East.

5000 BC
First ships on the Mediterranean Sea.

3500 BC
First cities spring up.

3300 BC
The Sumerians invent writing.

2100 BC
Exhausted British builders finish off Stonehenge.

1080 BC
Kite flying takes off in China.

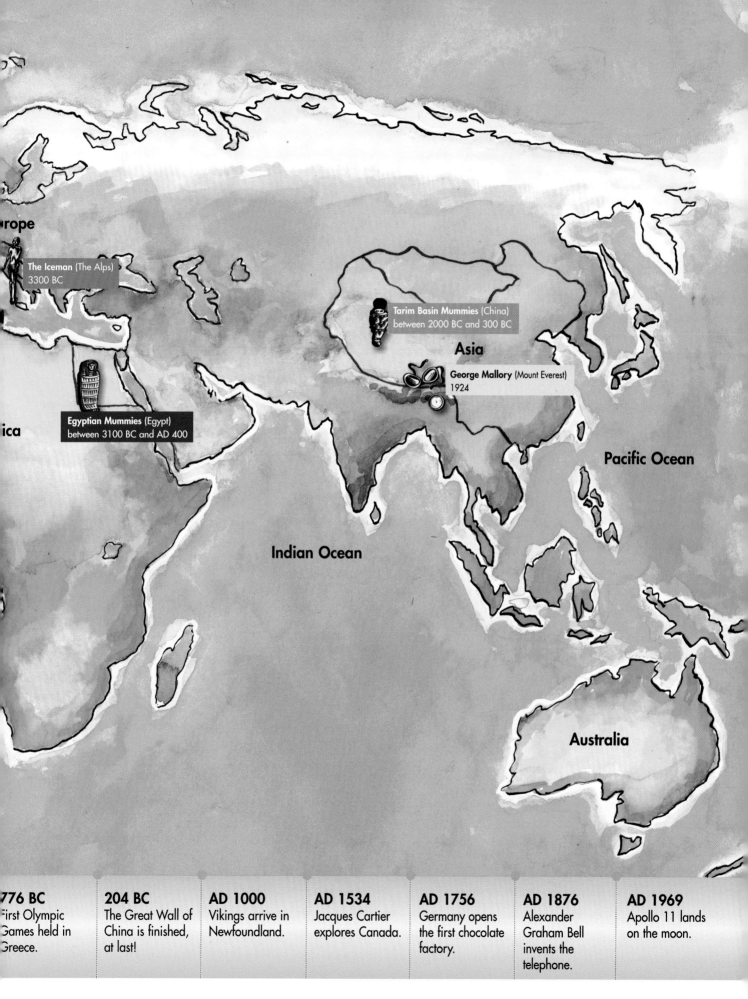

Europe

The Iceman (The Alps)
3300 BC

Tarim Basin Mummies (China)
between 2000 BC and 300 BC

Asia

George Mallory (Mount Everest)
1924

Egyptian Mummies (Egypt)
between 3100 BC and AD 400

Africa

Pacific Ocean

Indian Ocean

Australia

776 BC	204 BC	AD 1000	AD 1534	AD 1756	AD 1876	AD 1969
First Olympic Games held in Greece.	The Great Wall of China is finished, at last!	Vikings arrive in Newfoundland.	Jacques Cartier explores Canada.	Germany opens the first chocolate factory.	Alexander Graham Bell invents the telephone.	Apollo 11 lands on the moon.

INDEX